Pulling at Straws

Marsha Michaels

authorHOUSE®

AuthorHouse™
1663 Liberty Drive
Bloomington, IN 47403
www.authorhouse.com
Phone: 1-800-839-8640

First published by AuthorHouse 5/5/2011

ISBN: 978-1-4567-3444-2 (e)
ISBN: 978-1-4567-3733-7 (sc)

Library of Congress Control Number: 2011905872

Printed in the United States of America

Any people depicted in stock imagery provided by Thinkstock are models,
and such images are being used for illustrative purposes only.
Certain stock imagery © Thinkstock.

This book is printed on acid-free paper.

Acknowledgements

I would like to thank my friend and mentor, Barbara Rose Brooker, who crossed my path when I took her Creative Writing class at Olli at San Francisco State University. A published author in her own right knew and understood my passion for having an untold story. She guided my dream with just the right words of inspiration that allowed me to find my own voice and put it to paper.

I want to thank my classmates for reading through the many drafts I sent them, and for their constant support, when they knew not where I was going.

I consider myself fortunate to have met and befriended all.

My friends and family, who muddled along with me, will go unnamed to protect them, know that I am grateful.

Thanks to Nancy Bosshard for editing the early drafts; a special thanks to Baby Jode and Kimberly for the final draft.

I want to thank all that participated in making my reality into a story with a social history. Your efforts were cutting edge. My heartfelt regret for your loss of years, while imprisoned for the lack of our government's judgment of what is criminal.

Finally, to my husband Alberto who is judgment-free of all my activities, past and present.

Table of Contents

Acknowledgements

I would like to thank my friend and mentor, Barbara Rose Brooker, who crossed my path when I took her Creative Writing class at Olli at San Francisco State University. A published author in her own right knew and understood my passion for having an untold story. She guided my dream with just the right words of inspiration that allowed me to find my own voice and put it to paper.

I want to thank my classmates for reading through the many drafts I sent them, and for their constant support, when they knew not where I was going.

I consider myself fortunate to have met and befriended all.

My friends and family, who muddled along with me, will go unnamed to protect them, know that I am grateful.

Thanks to Nancy Bosshard for editing the early drafts; a special thanks to Baby Jode and Kimberly for the final draft.

I want to thank all that participated in making my reality into a story with a social history. Your efforts were cutting edge. My heartfelt regret for your loss of years, while imprisoned for the lack of our government's judgment of what is criminal.

Finally, to my husband Alberto who is judgment-free of all my activities, past and present.

Altitude and Attitude

*E*verything started innocently enough. I remember buying an ounce of pot, weighing it for accuracy on the triple beam scale. Then I was asked to split it with a friend, bringing down our costs. Soon everybody wanted an ounce, so I bought a pound for about $200.00, and I broke it up into sixteen, one-ounce bags and sold them for $70.00 each. I was not handling the financial end. That would be Alan Diamond, my high school boyfriend; I was the saleswoman. At the time I was living in my hometown, in a nearby borough from where I was born. My place was located in the west village on Jane Street in New York City. I was only twenty-one, working for the May Company buying office. My boss was Dawn Mello, who became the president of Bergdorf Goodman years later. I held the position of Buyer for home furnishings fabrics. It was a man's business; I was cutting edge and told, very cute. The mini-dress was in full fashion at the time and I was a big supporter of this new dress style. I was well liked and successful with all my buyers who ranged from coast to coast. How I went from professional to the bohemian/hippy is quite the tale to tell.

Many, many years later I found myself flying into Denver at the request of the FBI to have a chat at their headquarters. I remember it was a cold day with snow on the streets. It had been years since I crunched along on icy sidewalks. The air was crisp and the sky was a true Colorado blue. The choice the FBI gave me had been either a casual Saturday informal meeting or a date with the Grand Jury. On the phone, these agents had sounded like thugs. But on my arrival, I discovered the agents were long hairs themselves. It was strange how I felt familiar with the lead prosecutor, who I later found out had been a defense attorney for drug dealers in Mendocino County, working the opposite side of the law. On the close of this grueling interrogation, he was amazed at how this smuggling operation had successfully gone on for so many years. He asked me, "Has anyone written a book on this intriguing story?" His question has always stayed with me. But I am getting ahead of myself.

After high school graduation, Alan attended the

University of Arizona, a party college. I went to work at Bloomingdales on 59th Street and attended classes at New York School of Interior Design. We both dated others, but kept in close touch. When my father died at the young age of forty-seven, Alan flew back to see me. He had this way of hopping on planes. Buying a cheap ticket from Tucson to Phoenix. Then the plane went on to New York City. He would pretend to be asleep; and once the plane was airborne to his actual destination, he would play to the stewardess that he slept through his ticket stop. He had family in New York. He would negotiate a free return ticket, giving him a few days to visit. This was the story he told me; I asked no details.

I was certain that there was romance between us. We were each other's first love. I was fourteen when we had our first date. It was a fraternity party at his home. I met his parents that first night. Both were immigrants from Vienna with thick accents. Not until much later did I learn their story of escaping the Nazi regime.

While Alan was exploring out west, I met a nice Jewish boy at work. Marvin was a red-haired jokester. I hate jokesters! He treated me well, took me out to many nice places, we fell into regular dating, leading to a faux type of engagement. Our couple friends were planning weddings; "how about you two?" was easily asked of us. There were a few problems in partnering. Marvin's father was a Cantor, the singer for a Rabbi.

3

If we married, we would be expected to keep a Kosher home. My grandparents kept a Kosher home, but were lax for the grandchildren's needs, my aunt recently informs me just forty years later!

But Marvin ate bacon every weekend. Was he really going to change for his parents, who resided three states away? I was having what I now call a "lulu" moment, getting frustrated, but going with the flow.

Marvin and I took a road trip to see his parents. It was about a four-hour drive, for some reason I insisted on driving his new Volkswagen Bug. We were on the New Jersey turnpike. He complained I was tailgating. Before I knew it, I had caused quite the crash, mating with the front car. The Bug was badly wounded, but drivable. Insisting I continue driving when Marvin took the reins and let me have it. He said, "We will not discuss this with my parents."

"Fine with me", I retorted. I was really quite indifferent about the whole thing. When we arrived and introductions were made, my immediate impression was what a cold, conservative family. The home was dark, lifeless, and that included the conversation as well.

In comparison to the experience in my home, my parents would sit together in one club chair when there were two and had an attitude that if you wanted to make love swinging from a chandelier, go for it. If the participants were married, that is...

A few weeks later, deciding to drop a note to Alan, telling him of my engagement plans; that very next weekend, he showed his smiling tan face at my door. His hair was longer than usual and his attitude playful. "Getting married, eh?"

"Oh I don't know", I say, "probably." After we had caught up, he said, "I have something for you to try." We were sitting in my very small, cramped living room on my pullout couch when he lights up, not a Marlboro but a joint.

"Here just take a few sips."

"Hmmm, I'm afraid."

"Why?" he asks, "Trust me, you're safe."

Indeed I was. Needless to say the faux engagement with Marvin was instantly over as the romance with Alan blossomed once again.

Now I'm out on the streets selling pot to many of my vendors. It was innocent enough and fun watching the ordinary conservative men getting high in their offices, and then heading out to their martini lunches.

"Make sure you never tell my wife," many said to me.

I would pack up six ounces a day in my Mother's hand-me-down Bottega Veneto handbag and return home with more cash income than I made in a forty-hour week at my job.

As our relationship flourished, Alan suggested

I move out to Aspen Colorado, where we could live together and explore an entirely different lifestyle. It caused quite a dilemma to leave my professional life, reside outside the tri-state area that no one in my family had attempted to leave since the immigration of my grandfather from Palestine. This was not going to be welcome news to my family.

I found myself walking around the same six blocks for an inordinate amount of time, minutes maybe! I found myself ringing the bell where Alan was staying with his brother and live-in girlfriend.

"That's my girl," he says to Irene.

"How do you know?"

"It's destiny, meant to be."

Weeks later I got up the nerve to reveal to my mother the exciting news. Joey, as my Dad called her, and I were to meet at the 57th Street Hamburger Hamlet for lunch and a chat.

Remembering back after Dad's passing, Mom went to work for the family business, fine jewelry manufacturer. It was close to four years later and she was putting her young life back together.

Joey and I weren't as close as one might think, as she always let Dad answer my questions, which led to a very special relationship between the two of us. When I did tell Mom my latest plans on moving, I casually mentioned that Alan and I smoked pot together. It was probably not the best timing. Joey was telling me how one must cut back their portions as we age to keep trim. I at the time was 105 pounds so her conversation did not hold much reality for me. Forgetting to ask for the other half of her meal to go, Mom was instantly terrified and certain I would be shooting heroin that very night.

As I mentioned, it wasn't that Alan was some stranger to my parents. We dated all through high school and never got in trouble (that they knew of). After Dad's passing, Alan's mother came to show respect while Mom sat "Shiva" (a Jewish tradition honoring the dead.)

We were young and adventurous; but did not know what was in store for me. My mother was never one to ask for details once I came of age, and that was a blessing.

Thinking Mom had made peace with my decision, I received an unexpected phone call from my Uncle, Mom's brother.

"Hi doll face, let's meet for lunch. Mom says you have some new plans."

"Ok, set it up", I reply.

Seated, he begins with, "What can I do to keep you here with your widowed Mother? How about a nice European vacation, all expenses paid?" With no appetite I listened to his offerings and temptations.

Thinking to myself, he has got to be out of his mind. His sister is dating, building a new life. I had already moved out, living with a girlfriend. After five years, her widow weaves were in the back of the closet.

When it was apparent that the negotiation was going nowhere, I reminded my uncle that his sister, at twenty-two, ran off to Louisiana to marry my father against her own father's wishes as my father was leaving for England and WW2. I marched myself out of that very exclusive restaurant and took a sixty-seven block walk to inform my mother that I too was twenty-two and leaving to see some of the world. And yes, I would be "living in sin" as defined by that generation.

Everyone in the family and many close friends thought that if Dad hadn't died, this would not be happening. In secret, Mom realized that this child of hers had a special bond with her father. I had him for only seventeen years, but the legacy he left me was a lifetime of lessons. Most of all, I witnessed his warmth, his daily affection and how he was a lover to both his girls.

With his spirit, I packed with confidence and headed west....

Living High

The plane was banking in to land at the Denver Airport. I had just witnessed the Rocky Mountains looming below, all green, gold and snow-capped. With a huge sigh, I had made it. I thought to myself, I could die now. Crazy I know, but it was a tendency I had when I accomplished a great goal or overcame a challenge. It was this insecure habit I had of never feeling capable.

Alan was waiting breathlessly for all the electronics I was bringing for the music collection he had begun. Just as I am no techie, reel-to-reel in its day was also a mystery. With everything collected and loaded into the truck, we headed for our new home.

Crossing over the Vail Pass, the first of several high mountain passes, on the way to Aspen, Alan pulled into a scenic lookout so I could take in the scope of this glorious looking state. I only had the Adirondacks of New York to compare and trust me there was no contest. When we pulled over, with the dryness of the air (along with a little herbal smoke), my body was feeling heavy, especially my legs, I felt myself buckling over. Alan assured me it was the altitude and my body would adjust in a day or so. After about five hours, we arrived in Pitkin County and drove directly to our first home, a small one-bedroom apartment. It was newly constructed, clean with a park in front and it sat a few blocks from the bottom of the famous Ajax Mountain.

At dawn the next day, I stood up on the bed to look out the horizontal window that gave me a glimpse of my new surroundings. I was childlike, enthralled by the wonder of this place, something so brand new and beautiful.

As we headed out for our first walk around town, I realized I was looking behind as I learned to do living in a city. Alan told me, "There is no need to do that here." No need to be worried about being robbed or jumped from behind. I always found that remark naive, as there are crazies everywhere. But, in time, I realized it was about as safe as one could find.

After the initial day of getting settled, decorating in the style of cheap chic and buying our very first plant, a fuchsia, I was amazed at how quickly I adapted to mountain life. Once Alan began taking me around meeting his friends, I couldn't imagine what adventures might be in store for me. Everyone I met came from different parts of the country. From the southern drawl of Tennessee, to the mid-west of Chicago, California, Boston, just to name a few, what was it that drew so many to this little spot on the planet? It was a migration of longhaired hippies (the clean types). Some were fleeing the Vietnam draft. Many found they came to escape the headlines of what exactly our country was doing. The major newspapers were the enemy. For the most part, everyone I met was seeking a better life. Smoking dope was the norm and so was healthy outdoor living. Smoking pot did not make you tired and lazy, just the opposite. We would hike the trails for hours, camping in sublime areas only 4-wheel drive vehicles were able to reach. For me, I had never been camping before, so that was an adventure I recall with delight. The closest I came to such outings was being a Brownie and Girl Scout. This activity was a step up or should I say a giant leap from fashionable high heels to a pair of hiking boots from J.C. Penny.

Who would have thought that camping, getting high, pondering life (as I knew it) would open up my mind to the world? The sky's Little and Big Dippers, faces and scenes with animals in the clouds. "Look, do you see the elephant passing in that cloud?" There was much laughter and story telling, youth in the making. A far cry from the outside world, now consumed with killing resulting from the fear mongering of the "domino theory." All I could tell was, I found bliss in this outer edge of peace, love and a judgment free society. If this was the true hippy movement, I had found a new home.

Often thinking of my mother in New York City eating her half portions, I developed quite an appetite for cooking and dining. Always a nauseating picky eater, a couple of puffs of Colombian Gold cleared that condition up immediately.

After my first smoke back in New York, I took Alan to a neighborhood restaurant ordering an eggplant specialty. The taste of the dish was orgasmic and it led me to the full passion of the culinary life.

Dealing with high altitude cooking I learned some interesting lessons. Never have a dinner party where I would be serving Cornish game hen, for the first time. One of our guests was a chicken connoisseur. George was licking his chops with the smells coming from the kitchen, just three feet away. Unfortunately, it never occurred to me that cooking time was longer in high altitude than at sea level. Surprises make for a good article in life's lessons, particularly in the gourmet world. I was a novice so I just kept watching those baby hens take their time. Close to two hours in, I decided that the hens were communicating with me; smoking pot can do that to you, (just kidding!). However, I made the decision, or perhaps a deal, for the meal to be great; it was and I vowed to never cook another hen again and I haven't.

Once a butcher shop opened in town, preparing meals became much easier. Remembering walks with Rachel, my maternal grandmother, she would tell me, "Your butcher should be your best friend." Besides telling you how to prepare and for how long and at what temperature, cooking was the way to your man's heart. I just love those classic lines to this day, doesn't everyone? Who out there doesn't take pleasurable whiffs at onions and garlic sautéing away when entering a warm, cozy home?

It wasn't long after my big move before Alan and I met Nils, a six -week-old Irish setter puppy. Just another ordinary day, if you can call it that. He was the last of the litter; our names were tattooed on this puppy's head. We bought him right there in a hardware store. Not like today's adoptions, he was first carried, and then allowed to walk right next to us. By the time we made it home, we were all bonded!! Nils was loyal and courageous. Within a month, he broke his puppy leg while running next to the kids on the bunny slope at the ski mountain.

After the cast was fitted, he was right back out there, ever loyal to the children.

Leash laws and discipline were all but forsaken. Nils was arrested numerous times by the animal control for being off leash and hanging out at the back of restaurant kitchens. Perhaps he suffered with the munchies from second hand smoke! He was a trotter all his life. When the fines started peaking at $100, an outrageous amount of money, I would go to court and plead for mercy.

"You know judge, Setters are loony. Perhaps a light slap on the hand would be wishful thinking."

I would run into Judge Tim, a friend when not in his robes. But in court we got little mercy. Who would have thought back then this experience of puppy testifying was a practice run for a more serious circumstance in years to come?

Alan and I needed to move out of the apartment and found a great side-by-side duplex with a nice yard. An enclosed yard was the answer to our mounting court fines for Nils. The structure itself, an original, was woody with a character all its own. This was the first time I actually lived in a house. I grew up in apartments never knowing the luxury of home living. There were many applicants wanting to rent half the duplex, but Alan simply went directly to the owner's daughter, handing her six one hundred dollar bills. "This should cover first and last" he said.

"Oh," she responds, "An easy transaction; just two nice folks and a puppy." We moved right in that day. The lesson: cash talks!

Winter was coming, my first living in the mountains. The ski slopes were opening. I had some rather frightening experiences skiing in Vermont, so I was leery to give it a go. Alan explained I could take ski lessons, GLM, the graduated ski method. With this approach, one starts on two-foot skis, no poles. The next day three foot, ad poles, and then up to the recommended ski length for one's height. He assured me the Rocky Mountain snow was completely different from the ice in the East. I recall literally taking off my skis and walking down the mountain on my last skiing episode years before. Remembering the horrific bodily pain I suffered, plus the physical and mental danger of being hit by another skier, it had been a nightmare!!

In truth, the Aspen slopes were so wide that on one mountain range one can literally ski for a mile before having to make a turn. I liked that. Also, on a sunny day there was a dry cold, not the bitter cold as I was use to back on the East Coast. So this is why everyone has a ski tan. I was becoming more convinced by the day.

Skiing was so much easier than I had anticipated. In no time, I could ski, not black diamonds, but a nice blue trail, a beginning intermediate. It was February 13th, not a Friday. "Alan, I said, "let's go, it's a perfect day."

The weather and snow conditions were at peak. He was more than happy that I was becoming sport-oriented. Alan was a true sportsman. He played ball, skied, was frequently glued to sports on TV, (especially the New York Yankees, which I always felt was his true love.)

On that day, our friend Nancy and her friend Spence, a ski instructor, joined us. Spence was going to help me ski steep moguls, and I was ready. But when my bindings kept releasing, without any safety consciousness, I clamped them down tightly. At the very first challenging mogul I planted that pole; but, my left leg was stiff, it would not allow me to make the turn. Turning left had always been difficult. I never knew why I fell. Then, came the sound of breaking bones....

I went down in slow motion just as all my falls have been. I remember seeing Nancy and Alan looking down from the ski lift above, what Nancy repeated to me later was, "Oh no, that's a terrible accident!" and Alan replied, "That's our girl."

The Ski Patrol was there almost immediately. I was in no pain; that meant I was somewhat comatose. As the patrol worked on my one leg, securing it for the toboggan ride down, I started screaming.

"What the hell," I hear.

"Shit could it be her other leg?" After a minute I am told the other leg needed to be bound as well.

I was so out of it. I did not have a clue that having both legs bound wasn't normal.

My biggest fear came when they said, "Ok, are we ready for the trip down the hill?" Instantly I thought of the movie, Spellbound, with Ingrid Bergman and Gregory Peck and the lines, the ski lines. I remembered an "out of control scene".

Once again the dealmaker side of me comes out, let me be safe. Since this might be my last trip down the mountain. I enjoyed the sun on my face, asking one of the ski patrol guys if perhaps they had a little smoke for me.

Domesticity & Recovery

I left the hospital after much fuss about possibly having bones broken in both legs. X-rays showed major break of the right femora and the left ankle. After the surgery, which included pins and plates, my once lovely legs looked like Frankenstein and Fred Munster's head. This, the best orthopedic doctor in the Valley was no cosmetic surgeon. I managed to make the record of most broken bones in one fall that season. Frankly it never occurred to me that the scars wouldn't fade. My main concern was walking again. Like many other sufferings I endured, there was my Mother's voice reminding me "this too shall pass". I appeared to be racking up burdens to bear. Perhaps it was a pre-destiny exercise in what was to come.

Thankfully the new duplex was on ground level and

very manageable with the use of a silver walker. I was in the beginning stages of my "Yin Yang" education. A life of balance was the goal. I started practicing Buddhist theories without being a Buddhist. It was the "in" thing to do.

What was disconcerting was that Alan had to leave town for several weeks to do "business". Luckily I had several friends that could help me out, as driving was not an option.

Additionally, I didn't realize there would be painful muscle spasms and then there was that itch inside the full leg cast.

Alan reminded me to just have a smoke, as if that was the fix-it drug. Surprisingly, it was! The spasms would stop. It's an herb, Monkey Face, he would say. "Monkey Face" was his nickname for me. It came from yet another movie starring Cary Grant and Joan Fontaine. Sometimes I thought we were characters in a movie.

Nancy, originally from Southern California, was quick to my rescue with a knitting needle that took care of the itch. She also brought a new arrival, Tamara, from Santa Barbara, California, who would become another one of my life-long friends.

When we first met, I was sitting in the backyard throwing yet another tennis ball into Nil's mouth.

Tamara was light-hearted and fancy-free. I soon found out she was a cowboy lover. If Dale Evans were a blond, this would be her, riding off into the sunset with the "Roy Rogers" pick of the week.

Besides all the folly, Tamara became my constant companion during my recovery. With Alan away doing a "deal," she would stop by daily with whatever was needed. We would hang out in the yard on lounge chairs, tanning ourselves looking up at the beautiful mountains, music playing while she taught me how to embroider. All my California girlfriends did crafts. Never once back east, except for holding my arms out for Grandma as she made yarn into balls, did anyone do crafts.

I learned candle making, macrame and now embroidery. Tamara was working on a piece de resistance. It was a project embroidering a marijuana plant on the jean leg of her latest cowboy flirtation. Now that was very cool.

I could not begin to even draw the plant, so Tam stenciled it all for me on the leg of Alan's jean and the project began.

At times I would wonder if she were secretly hired to care for me.

The answer was obvious when, one day she walked in to put groceries away and found me crawling with a Pledge can and rag, dusting the house. I would throw the Pledge around the room, and then crawl to the specified area and clean. If Tamara were on the payroll, one would think she would have put a stop to my craziness. Instead, we just together had a great laugh, then and now....

When Alan returned, many weeks later, he and I began walking together for what is now called physical therapy. Each step was excruciatingly painful. After the cast was removed, my legs were shrunken and hairy. The only good thing was my upper body was in tiptop shape as it did double the work since my lower extremities were compromised.

Alan was patient.

"Will I ever be able to walk normally?" I would ask him.

"Absolutely Monkey Face, it just takes time."

Tears would stream down my face.

"How about we head for a trip down to the Caribbean and meet up with friends in Jamaica?"

"Really, can we afford that?"

"You don't need to worry about finances", and off we went.

On arrival to this tropical paradise, friends met us with cheers and open arms. They too were worried how I would recoup. The hard part came as I stepped onto the sand. If I thought cement was agonizing, this was more then a match.

After two months, I was not only recovered but had begun looking into starting a little import business of batik textiles. We had toured the plant and I knew this fashion was cutting edge. It was an improvement over "tie dye." Back home I set up "Blue Mountain Designs" after the famous coffee. I purchased enough fabric sampling to bring back and make into dresses by a seamstress. Embroidering was the end of crafting; I was more into the business aspect.

All the trips Alan and I took to other countries, such places as Jamaica and Colombia, I always brought something back. From South America, the hand-woven mantas were my biggest success. Friends would buy up my samples before I was able to begin marketing. In the end, importing laws and duties were such a hardship, good ideas and intentions fell by the wayside.

Back home in the Rockies, the slopes were closing, the rains were starting and the locals were attending to business.

There was something in the wind, quiet chats, with our group of men only.

They no longer used the house phone, but would find public phones at weird hours of the night.

Buzz....

A load was coming.

(What the hell did that mean?)

Setting up Shop

*I*t was a whiteout. Snow coming down in such force, no one could see anything, let alone a truck loaded with pot pulling into the driveway. Before I knew what was happening, my very groovy walk-in closet was stacked with strange bricks of weed, moldy, pungent and green. Immediately we started unwrapping packages, evaluating cost. Pretty, like California pot, it wasn't! But this was before horticulturists got involved. This was "dirt weed" from Mexico and it smoked just fine. We started cleaning the sticks and seeds out of the kilos; after all no one likes to pay for excess weight. From hours of cleaning, we could see in the mirror we were all covered with green dust. Could this be the "greening of America"?

On the outside, there was a raging war in Vietnam.

Where as our clan was a far cry from the killing, destruction and the imperialism that was rampant in our country, I felt proud to be part of a peaceful movement.

It was the birth of an entire new industry; everyone was working.

The smugglers, buyers, sellers, truckers, carpenters (building secret compartments in vehicles), along with marijuana cleaners, and one of my favorites, the house hunters were fully employed. There was never a doubt the product produced a high. It was not yet becoming acknowledged that marijuana also brought comfort to many suffering from diseases, as well as bringing about the best generation of music in history.

I was employed as the house hunter along with several other young women. Our employers were our "old' men." (boyfriends) It was a family business. As more loads of pot were scheduled, different locations were set up across the country. A few gals would load up their trunks with samples weighing one hundred pounds and head across country to set up a "stash" house. It was a distribution point where buyers could come to make purchases to bring back to their individual territory. I would describe us as jobbers in the early years. The middleman from the smuggler to the retailer is a good comparison. Almost instantly there were hundreds involved in these dealings. College campus became a stronghold of supply and demand, a perfect fit for distributing the product. The country was at the height of discontent with our leaders. History played out, as witnessed by Kent State.

Business was booming. No one should think real work wasn't being done here. Marijuana never crippled creativity, intelligence or inventiveness. If anything, there was more ingenuity involved than one would imagine.

Road trips turned into folklore.

Two of the girls left the Rockies with a full trunk, only to run into complications in Kansas. An unexpected snowstorm, early in the season, created dangerous driving conditions. No one wanted a spin out, especially with a load of pot.

The girls pulled into a hotel to wait it out. Martin Luther also was in their company. He had to be sneaked in as "NO DOGS" was posted. He was a large black standard puddle who walked with the grace and stature much like his owner. In the middle of the night, he became ill. With the help of the night crew at the hotel, who were sworn to secrecy, he was rushed to an emergency animal hospital. He was suffering an epileptic seizure. He survived. Within a day or so, they were all back on the road again safe, sound and delivered.

Some road trips led to awakenings outside of the

business of transportation. When I first saw the city that was to be my home of the future. Elizabeth and I were traveling on California Interstate 101 with our spare tire in the back seat. In order to carry double the quantity of product in the trunk, this was necessary but only for a short distance to where we were unloaded. Then we headed toward Sausalito, not knowing where we were. Elizabeth was crossing lines sporadically, looking for the right exit, when we heard and saw the frightening flashing red lights of the Highway Patrol. She looked at me and said, "Stay cool, I will take care of this." We had forgotten to put the tire back in the trunk. With frantically beating hearts, the cop approaches, glances at the tire, when Eliza jumps out of the car and starts to chat it up about being lost, which we were. The cop, more than suspicious says, "Ma'am, open the trunk." The pop of the trunk reverberated. To his utter surprise, the trunk was vacuumed clean. That cop was so disappointed we thought he would get out a magnifying glass looking for a seed. Fortunately for us, one cannot be arrested for a strange odor. That night I stood on the Sausalito pier looking toward the bright lights of San Francisco. Silently I said to myself, "I am going to live here someday."

I was sure I had an herbal (marijuana) spirit that protected me through some of the most bazaar situations. One afternoon driving through the Poconos, a mountain range in Pennsylvania, I was speeding when it was my turn to pull over to the blaring sounds of police sirens. Two of us were in a large rental car with a huge trunk that was fully loaded.

'What's your rush little lady?"

"Oh officer, hi, we are headed home with our animals and just not paying attention to the speed on the downhill."

"Those are fine looking dogs you got there"

"Thanks, they are really like our children."

"How far east are you headed?"

"To see family in New York."

"Ok, well you drive safe now, wish you were staying the night; I would love to take you out for dinner."

On the slow pull out, with a smile and a wave, we howled; the dogs joined in as well.

Over the decade of the 1970's, "The Biz" (as it was now known), flourished and became more sophisticated. As the years sped by, there was much more caution as the FBI was beginning to investigate what had evolved into a huge surge of marijuana sales along with who was behind it.

My last and most memorable assignment was to find an estate outside the Boston area. It had to be adaptable for absolute privacy. I knew what was coming was on a different scale entirely. I never had the details but my ears were perked. Alan always felt the less I knew would protect him as well as myself in case there was a bust.

After a few days touring various rentals, I found the perfect Colonial home situated on a one hundred acre estate with a mile long curving driveway leading through a dense wooded forest. Better than anticipated we were thrilled with the setting. It was a glorious fall that year, with New England in full dazzling colors. The smells were intoxicating. As I walked through the woods, my right eye went blurry. Like a cold wind chilled the eye; but the vision would remain unclear. There was much to do getting decorated and setting up home for the six individuals who would be occupying the residence. This was a dream home come true for me. The rent blew us away; this much space for $500.00 a month! It was a project that put my design eye to work. Since our time there would be short, just to years end; I went into thrifty decor. The mansion was true Colonial, wood floors and paneling, high ceilings. The surrounding towns were full of antique and thrift stores. Estate sales took my breath away.

We collected the finest silverware, English bone china, velvet couches, armoires, mirrors, lace, and linens. Everything was dirt-cheap.

October quickly ran into November, favorite holidays of the harvest were fast approaching. We were all happy, full of life, feeling immortal and generally stoned as we gathered maple leaves to dry for the centerpiece for our dining room table-adding pumpkins, gourds, and huge displays of mums in every color possible. We located the best markets for the feast that would be prepared by all. Our dining room was formal, including a bell on the floor that the one sitting at the head could press and the make believe butler would be called to serve. It was a riot.

We all gathered for the harvest, the turkey with all the traditional trimmings of chestnuts and sausage, apples, raisins, wild rice, fresh cranberry, green beans with walnuts, fig balsamic, breads and pies assorted to meet everyone's taste. I thought dressing as pilgrims would be fun, but did not get support from the men. We ladies dressed up and looked as though we were right off the Mayflower ship. The harvest was a huge success and in the shadows, somewhere on the one hundred acres of land, one of the biggest marijuana deals was taking place. I heard that thousands of kilos arrived packaged in blue paper.

There was no need for cleaning, as the quality was excellent. Gold Colombian they called it...later songs were written about this legendary product.

"The load" was orchestrated and moved out, all across the country, in record time. No region was missed. I would bet every smoker in that era tasted that peppery spice flavor that many to this day laugh over the "blue bricks." They showed up everywhere. Millions of dollars were made in a few months, but much more was lost. Not until later, many years later.

The winds were blowing and my eye was still blurry. I saw an ophthalmologist, who treated the condition with steroids. The treatment was successful, temporarily. It never occurred to me I might have something very seriously wrong. That too came years later.

We had bought so many valuable treasures in Massachusetts during our short stay, that this time we decided to ship everything back home in some of the moving vans at our disposal. "The gig," as it would be called, was over. Leaving the area left me with a heavy heart...

Departure

Returning to Aspen, we continued to live modestly in a rented cabin on the Roaring Fork River. It was another charmer with a huge deck. For me, there is nothing more soothing then the swirling & gushing of movement that a river makes. It is harmony to my soul.

After the blue brick deal was over the three partners went their separate ways with their individual millions in cash. One bought a ranch, another a home, all in different parts of the Valley. Alan and I decided perhaps it was time to put down permanent roots, build a custom designed home, on acreage that he had previously bought, and remain living in Aspen. We would no longer be downtown, which I did enjoy as I could walk to early morning yoga classes in a park two blocks away. After my daily yoga, an easy walk to Main Street for coffee with friends; then once I returned to work, all the boutiques where I was employed were also within walking distance. Never did it occur to me how grateful I should be for these 'walks'....

When the house project began to be discussed, I thought this project would fulfill a desire to further exercise my design skills. I was not able to spread my wings working with clothing and shoes. When I had the opportunity to work at an antique vintage shop, I learned much more about Art Deco and Art Nouveau from Eve, the owner. Now I was moving closer to my passion in home design.

All my experiences were for a reason. Did I know that at the time? Somewhat, perhaps in the back of my mind....

I was anxious to build. I was also aware that Alan had no intention of leaving the marijuana business behind. He would make no excuses for his choice of lifestyle. The excitement, the adventures, and the money—nothing could compare. I, on the other hand, felt the thrill was gone and it was time to get serious about "Real Work." My opinion was dismissed.

If we were to build, I would be in charge of everyday operations, as Alan would be away for weeks on end doing business. A black cloud hung over the property. The history of this particular valley was couples for whatever reason all broke up after settling in. Alan and I had close to ten years of living together in addition to our early dating years.

We threw caution to the wind and broke ground...

It was a winter build; one of the first with an arboretum through the center of the roof to provide what was then solar energy. Our builder was a furniture maker. He built this home with numerous custom details we would never have thought of ourselves. He was a purist with the woods he used, whether it was interior or exterior doors, cabinets, or shelves, nothing had an angle edge. Everything rolled like a magnificent yacht, dug in to the foundation and surrounded by a huge foundation wall. An artisan from California built the fireplaces. Nothing was a façade, rock upon rock with a special niche forming a marble seat where I would sit and rest my arm while enjoying the warmth of a fire.

The venture always seemed somewhat make believe. But it was real enough when business deals fell through and cost kept spiraling. For example, even though an entire mock-up was done the kitchen was wrong for me in its final stage. It was designed for a left-handed person. I wasn't, but Alan was.

We managed a year in the house together. We went through a Thanksgiving with not much joy. The kitchen worked fine, but I never connected personally with the project. It was just too big; I like cozy. I would have to wait another seven years in that far off place where I once recognized, "I could live there".

We could not keep this relationship together even though I could successfully duplicate any cover of a gourmet magazine for dinner on any night. In happier times, we would kid each other and say, "Ten years with any one man was long enough". Apparently, we had chosen different roads.

The move came swiftly as this was something that was underlying for at least a few years. We both suffered with mixed emotions but the reality was obvious for both of us. While I packed up years of history, he stayed away from the house. There was literally too much sadness. I remember Billy Holiday was playing on the stereo all the time.

Once I had found a new home with his help in Santa Barbara, California, he drove me to my new destination....

Diagnosis

When I was nineteen, I remember I began to have this urgency to pee at the most awkward times. Before a good night kiss, I would think, quick, kiss me so I can get upstairs to the bathroom. I convinced myself it was nervousness. Naturally at this young age, I shared this dilemma with no one. Always being an extremely nervous child, mother would blame Dad's side of the family. Years of throwing up on my way to school, this new occurrence was just another ailment in my repertoire.

What was most disconcerting was like the blurry eye; the urgency to pee would come and go.

Later, while living in the Rockies, it became apparent that any time I got over-heated the eye would go out. I could be playing tennis, taking a hot bath.

Then after moving to Santa Barbara, the heat would affect my balance. Once I was a good dancer. Now I could barely follow, tripping over myself. Forget closing my eyes, I completely lost balance.

I would track the symptoms. I knew it was electrical, my nervous system. With very little knowledge, I had this overwhelming feeling I had multiple sclerosis. I cannot tell you why I thought this except for one profound situation that led me to these thoughts.

I was working as a "Shop At Home Consultant" for a department store in Santa Barbara when I got a call to help a young woman with decorating her room in her family's house. When I met her I found she could not walk normally or speak clearly. She told me she had multiple sclerosis. She had suffered a severe exacerbation and had to leave her position as a judge's assistant. She moved back home with her family to be cared for. She touched me to the core. Instinctively I knew she was my mirror. After chatting with her I decided it was time to take all my little sensations to a doctor, again. My mother took me when I first had symptoms I was twenty; the doctors could find nothing. This diagnosis I heard over and over. The conversation would go, "What can I do for you?" After sharing my self-diagnosis and symptoms the professional looked into my eyes and said, "Nope, no M.S. here." As a sidebar, I later found out, the doctors all looked for a cloudy optic nerve, which has never showed itself.

By this time, I was dating a much younger man from Argentina, who needed a green card and was pursuing me intently. Why not marry him? I was always a bit outside the law. I certainly knew nothing was forever. Besides twelve, thirteen years my junior, men wed younger women all the time.

It was at this point I received a job opportunity, which would require I make a move. Santa Barbara became a five-year transition from Colorado to the city I already knew was a perfect fit, San Francisco.

After the settling in process, we found ourselves walking and biking up and down the hills (with no helmets!). I started exercising at a local club, pumping iron when suddenly on one very hot day, I could barely move. I quickly found an air-conditioned restaurant and recovered, but not before the judge's assistant loomed large in my memory. I too was walking like a drunk....

Within that first year in San Francisco I turned forty and by then my left leg would not lift enough to clear the sidewalk. I kept tripping and, frankly, decided that I was finally in a metropolitan city, I could get a more accurate diagnosis and help from specialists.

At first I went to see an orthopedic doctor. I told him my symptoms and my personal diagnosis, again. He said, "Let's see, close your eyes, lift one leg." I could not without falling over. Oh my God, I do have M.S. You need to see a neurologist he suggested. All these years and this one professional orders one simple test, that no one else knew to perform?

The next week I got in to see a neurologist. He ordered an MRI, which was new technology. I had no expectation. Not really knowing the prognosis of this disease, I would have been happy with a diagnosis at last.

My cousin was in the medical field and chose not to tell me exactly what would happen in the prep for the screening. Knowing how panicky I was, it was probably for the best. Once I was strapped down, my head was clamped into a device. This was starting to feel like it was more than I bargained for. When I was inserted into the moving tube I began to panic. Someone was talking to me through the headphones, where I should have been listening to Rachmaninoff from the control booth. I made such a fuss, what if there is an earthquake? Who will pull me out of here? Realizing they had a very nervous patient, I was given an IV of Valium. That was much better. I was told it would be quite loud when the picture was being taken. I was finally relaxed enough to continue breathing and that the sound of jack hammering that lasted over 2 hours, eyes closed and extreme stillness, bothered me.

My new husband and cousin waited outside for moral support.

Everyone was very subdued about the outcome. I was told there was no cure, and multiple sclerosis was a progressive disease…

Dr. Deny my Neurologist, asked me several questions. "How fast were the symptoms happening?"

"Slowly, over years", I responded.

"Are you stiff or weak?"

"I think its stiffness."

"Does anything help when it happens?"

"Yes, absolutely, smoking pot."

"How long have you smoked and how often?"

"Every day for the last twenty years, unless I have a cold which is very rare."

Then with a big smile he said, "I see you found your own herbal remedy."

I waited for days before the results were in, thinking back on how everything happens for a reason, even being involved on the front lines of a marijuana smuggling operation.

When I got the call, I felt vindicated for what I always knew to be true. Later I would tell my family, as the scope of this disease you learn as you go. But for now, I rolled a little doob, prepared our favorite chicken cacciatore dish, and opened a nice Navarro Pinot Noir. Life was still good with more clarity.

Epilogue

*I*n 1983, when a ship traveling from Colombia to Mexico, loaded with thousands of pounds of pot, was busted off the coast of Cabo San Lucas. It was discovered riding low and dirty in the ocean by the Coast Guard. For whatever reason, the off loader (a smaller vessel) never met the ship to unload the product.

I was working communications with the Captain of the main ship. This was the second trip we had done together, the first being quite successful. It is still unknown if the off loader did not receive the proper co-ordinates to fulfill the mission.

The Coast Guard asked the Captain for permission to board. Philip, an ex-Marine, Special Forces, who served in Vietnam, knew to lay down arms and surrender. The newspapers reported this was the largest bust to have taken place, taking down a one hundred million dollar operation that had flourished for over a decade. The boat and the Captain's log were seized, and the Captain and his crew were taken to jail. All of the marijuana was burned.

When I left Aspen I thought I was done with drug dealing. But when my closest male friends approached me to take on this job, I was barely making ends meet and the pay they offered was decent. The job consisted of manning the phone for about six weeks as the boat made its way from Colombia to the coast of Mexico. Daily chats consisted of how good the fishing was and that was about it. On the other side of these calls were the partners awaiting the arrival of the shipment, who also checked in daily and I would report what was said. Everything was in code, the meaning of which I was not privy to.

In order to continue my regular job, I hired a friend to "phone sit" when I made design calls. We had all been part of the business in one- way or another throughout the years. Some folks were bi-lingual and helped with negotiations on price, quality and quantity. Others had capability for finding appropriate marinas to pull into, after business was done. Many took turns being part of the crew. All played backgammon and cards to pass the time.

At the time of the bust I was living with my soon to-be husband.

I received several thousand dollars and was told to leave town, thinking the FBI might be knocking on my door within hours.

No one was exactly thinking things through. Where was I going to go? I had a job and a life. Still I ended up calling a girlfriend and off we went to Big Bear for a week.

Just a little side story, I had been asked by the Captain, before the crew set sail for Colombia, if I would come down to Mexico and design the interior of the boat. This was exciting for me and I flew to where they were docked. Taking the shore tender out to the main vessel, the Federales stopped us inquiring if I was a "puta" (whore). With my typical indignation and a pointed finger, I replied,

"No soy ninguna puta" (I am no whore). "Soy el interiorista para esta nave" (I am the interior designer for this ship). Moving right along, I again felt terribly off balance. Trying to board the ship, I felt I could have fallen into the water at any time. Thankfully, one of the men extended a hand, an arm, and a body if I so desired....

After the diagnosis, a dozen years later, it all made sense.

I ordered the best wood blinds, all custom made

for the portholes and quality carpeting. Interestingly, I actually made more money doing the design work than what I wound up with after the bust.

After a week, we simply headed home and I went back to work.

The FBI never came to the apartment where the phone lines had been set up.

I took the position in San Francisco and my new husband and I moved there in 1985. Two years later, Alberto calls to me from the downstairs garage.

"Honey, the FBI is here to see you."

I greeted the two men and was served papers. They were now just getting around to investigating who were the "Kingpins in the 1983 bust; those who were behind the smuggling, the ones who made a great deal of money.

This was when I received that infamous invitation to fly into Denver and testify as to what I knew....

When I was at the FBI Headquarters, they began the interview by asking, "How did this all begin?"

My answers shall remain confidential. There were about eighty witnesses being interviewed. The FBI was able to gather enough information to make a case for a conviction locking these young men up for ten years.

Alan was also busted on an entirely different

smuggle, that came in by plane, around the same time the FBI informed me.

"I had heard that smuggle never happened."

"We have photographs," which they proceeded to show me. In addition, he was part of a sting operation, caught red handed so they said.

Another agent arrives and states, "I understand you lived with Alan Diamond for ten years. What can you tell us about his business?"

With a smile, I replied, "Not a thing. He never confided in me about his business dealings." And that was the truth....

Alan had been in contact with me and was concerned that I would be indicted, which I was not. Although he had married and had a child, my heart was broken, yet again.

In the corner sat a man representing the IRS.

I turned to him and said, "For your information, the monies I made were declared on my taxes as design work. You have no case against me." He lowered his head, hopefully in shame.

The lead prosecutor walked me out and said, "I really hope this wasn't to upsetting for you." "Are you kidding me," was my response. "I just spilled my guts on my friends and one time family members, for what?"

"They just wouldn't stop," he replied.

With a huge sigh of frustration, "Yeah, I know...."

The "boys" spent fortunes on lawyers, lost their homes, some their wives, and children lost years without their fathers. All were sent away from family and friends for years to various prisons. (Actually they were considered white-collar tennis camps).

In looking back, I see greed as the motivator, no different from what this country is dealing with today: the greed of politician's, the greed of Wall Street, in mortgage companies, banks, Ponzi schemes.

What I know for sure is that using taxpayer's money to warehouse (jail) these guys was a pure waste.

Why does my government need to be regulating mine or anyone else's recreational activity, and punishing those who supply what was in demand? I myself can now legally purchase all the medicinal marijuana I want, and I could buy for my friends, as I suspect many do with pot club cards. It is an outrageous hypocrisy.

I would like to know why some marijuana clubs have stairs to climb with no disability access? Why are there only two disability parking spaces in a large parking area?

Why one needs to stand in a long line, waiting his or her turn? It brings to mind what bread lines during the depression must have been like.

For all our sake, I ask my Federal government, can

we please legalize and validate benign marijuana as an important lucrative business opportunity?

It has now been twenty years since the diagnosis of multiple sclerosis. The disease has taken its progressive toll on me and I have made the necessary compromises. My walking is limited to maybe two blocks with the support of a walker. I can still drive, thankfully and use an electric scooter to get around.

I have endured this journey for forty plus years.

I still have my daily tokes; which eases the stiffness of my body like no other remedy.

I have to ask, "Is this really criminal?"

XXX

www.ingramcontent.com/pod-product-compliance
Lightning Source LLC
Chambersburg PA
CBHW020409290526
45785CB00005B/2482